HOW TO GET STARTED ON YOUR NURSING CAREER

I0139948

BY NEKESHA JOHNSON MSN, APRN, FNP-BC

CONTENTS

CHAPTER 1

WHY CHOOSE NURSING?

Nursing is a fulfilling and rewarding profession that provides a host of benefits to those who pursue it. It is a career that demands dedication and compassion but also offers the opportunity to make a real difference in people's lives. Although nursing school can be challenging, it remains a worthwhile pursuit due to the many benefits of being a nurse. Remembering why you became a nurse in the first place will help you succeed, flourish, and overcome any obstacles you may encounter along the way.

I chose to pursue a career in nursing because of job stability, the ability to positively impact someone's life, and the knowledge and skills to assist my family's health needs. Nursing has profoundly shaped and impacted my life, which is why I want to share my knowledge and encourage others to consider this excellent career. In this chapter, we will explore the many reasons why nursing is a great profession to pursue and the numerous benefits that come with it.

1. Rewarding Career

One of the most significant benefits of becoming a nurse is the opportunity to save lives and provide comfort to those in need. Nurses are on the front lines of patient care and play a crucial role in the healthcare system. They provide emotional support, administer medications, monitor patient progress, and coordinate care with other healthcare professionals.

Nurses form close relationships with their patients and families, which can be quite rewarding. Few careers allow people to see the impact of their work firsthand and witness their patients' progress and recovery. Nurses often go above and beyond their job duties to provide comfort and support during difficult times. They are compassionate, empathetic, and generally want to make a positive impact on the world. If you're looking for a career that allows you to make a difference in people's lives, nursing might be the perfect choice.

2. Job Stability and Security

Nurses are in high demand, and it's a profession that offers excellent job stability. One reason for this is the high demand for nurses in the healthcare industry. Nurses are needed to care for patients in hospitals, clinics, nursing homes, and other healthcare settings. According to the Bureau of Labor Statistics, the employment of registered nurses is projected to grow 6% from 2021 to 2031, faster than the average for all occupations![1] This means that there will be plenty of job opportunities for those pursuing a career in nursing.

Another reason why nursing offers job stability is the aging population. As people get older, they require more healthcare services, which leads to an increased demand for nurses. The Baby Boomer

[1] Bureau of Labor Statistics, U.S. Department of Labor, Occupational Outlook Handbook, Registered Nurses, at https://www.bls.gov/ooh/healthcare/registered-nurses.htm

generation, which makes up a significant portion of the population, is now entering retirement age, and they will require more healthcare services in the coming years. This will lead to an even greater demand for nurses and other healthcare professionals.

Additionally, the COVID-19 pandemic has highlighted the importance of nurses in the healthcare system. Nurses have played a critical role in caring for patients with COVID-19, and their contributions have been recognized and valued by the public. As a result, there is now a greater appreciation for the work that nurses do, which will likely lead to increased funding for healthcare and greater demand for nurses in the future. Overall, the combination of a growing and aging population, as well as increased recognition of the importance of nurses, make nursing a stable and secure career choice.

3. Financial Security

In addition to job stability, nurses are paid quite well. The average salary for a registered nurse in the United States is $75,330 as of May 2020. However, this is just an average, and the peak salary for nurses with advanced degrees and specialized skills can be much higher. For example, nurse anesthetists have a median annual wage of $189,190, and nurse practitioners have a median annual wage of $117,670. These higher salaries make nursing a financially rewarding career choice.

4. Job Flexibility

Due to its high demand and the need for nurses 24/7, nursing provides a great deal of flexibility when it comes to work schedules. Nurses can choose from various schedules that work for their individual needs, from full-time, part-time, or per diem. Additionally, nurses can select what time they work, including days, nights, or a mixture of the two. The length of shifts also varies, from 8-hour shifts to 12-hour shifts. With so many options, nurses are guaranteed to find a schedule that works for their personal life.

5. Variety of Work Situations

Nursing offers a variety of work environments to choose from, including hospitals, clinics, nursing homes, community centers, schools, and even patients' homes. From a fast-paced and exciting environment like the ER or ICU, or a slower-pace location like a research clinic, there's bound to be a location that appeals to everyone. Even seemingly unrelated fields like technology and the legal sector need nurses! This wide range of work settings allows nurses to find jobs that align with their interests and passions. The high demand for nurses also provides opportunities for trying different specialties and finding their niche within the field.

6. Programs Available Everywhere

Nursing programs are widely available across the United States, making it easy for anyone interested in pursuing a career in nursing to find a program that suits their needs. According to the American Association of Colleges of Nursing, there were over 3,000 nursing programs in the US as of 2021, including undergraduate and graduate degree programs, as well as diploma and certificate programs. This means that aspiring nurses have many options to choose from, including traditional in-person programs, online programs, and hybrid programs that combine both in-person and online learning. Furthermore, many nursing programs offer flexible scheduling options to accommodate students' personal and professional obligations. With so many options available, it's easier than ever to pursue a career in nursing and obtain the education and training needed to succeed in this rewarding profession.

7. Opportunity for Career Growth

Nursing offers numerous opportunities for growth, leadership, and higher education. With a career in nursing, individuals can pursue advanced degrees, such as a Master's or Doctorate in Nursing, which can lead to leadership positions and increased job flexibility. They can also specialize in a particular area of healthcare, such as critical care or oncology, which can lead to career advancement and increased earning potential. Nurses can also pursue leadership roles within their organizations, such as becoming a nurse manager, nurse educator, or clinical nurse specialist, which can provide opportunities for mentoring and guiding other nurses. Overall, nursing is a field that encourages growth and offers a wealth of opportunities for individuals looking to take their careers to the next level.

8. Excellent Benefits

Nursing is a profession that typically offers excellent benefits to its employees. Many healthcare organizations provide nurses with comprehensive health insurance, including medical, dental, and vision coverage, as well as retirement benefits such as 401(k) plans. In addition to these traditional benefits, many organizations offer additional perks to their nursing staff, such as tuition reimbursement, professional development opportunities, and wellness programs. These benefits not only help to attract and retain skilled nurses, but they also promote a healthy work-life balance and demonstrate a commitment to the well-being of employees. These perks make it an attractive career choice for individuals looking for long-term job security and financial stability.

In conclusion, nursing is a profession that provides a multitude of benefits to those who pursue it. It offers the opportunity to make a real difference in people's lives, with job stability, financial security, and various work situations to choose from. Nursing programs are widely available, making it easy for anyone interested in pursuing a career in nursing to find a program that suits their needs. The field also offers opportunities for career growth, leadership, and higher education. Additionally, nursing is a profession that typically offers excellent benefits to its employees. With so many positive aspects, nursing remains a fulfilling and rewarding career choice that offers a lifetime of opportunities.

CHAPTER 2

THE DIFFERENCE BETWEEN VARIOUS NURSING ROLES

Multiple nursing roles have emerged over time to meet the increasing complexity of the healthcare field. To provide the best possible care for patients, there is a need for these individualized and specialized roles, each with different educational requirements and job duties. From basic patient care to complex medical procedures and advanced diagnosis and treatment, the different nursing roles are essential to ensure patients receive the appropriate care they need to recover and maintain their health. From certified nursing assistants (CNAs) to nurse practitioners (NPs), we'll discuss the various roles within nursing to find your perfect fit.

Certified Nursing Assistants (CNAs)

Certified Nursing Assistants (CNAs) are entry-level healthcare professionals who provide basic patient care under the supervision of a licensed nurse, usually a Registered Nurse (RN) or Licensed Practical Nurse (LPN). They are an essential part of the healthcare team and typically work in nursing homes, hospitals, assisted living facilities, and other long-term care facilities.

As entry-level healthcare professionals, CNAs are responsible for providing basic patient care. This includes assisting with activities of daily living, such as bathing, dressing, and feeding patients, as well as monitoring patients' vital signs and reporting any changes to the nursing staff. CNAs also help to maintain a clean and safe environment for patients and may be responsible for transporting patients to and from different areas of the healthcare facility.

In terms of education requirements, most CNAs complete a state-approved training program that can be completed in as little as a few weeks. The program includes both classroom instruction and hands-on clinical training to prepare students for the demands of the job. After completing the training, CNAs must pass a competency exam to become certified in their state. Some CNAs may also be required to have a high school diploma or equivalent.

Licensed Practical Nurses (LPNs)

Licensed Practical Nurses (LPNs) are healthcare professionals who provide basic patient care under the supervision of a Registered Nurse (RN) or physician. They typically work in hospitals, nursing homes, clinics, and other healthcare settings.

While CNAs provide basic patient care and assist with activities of daily living, LPNs have a broader scope of practice that includes administering medication, monitoring vital signs, and performing basic medical procedures such as changing dressings or inserting catheters. Unlike CNAs, LPNs can administer medication and perform more advanced medical procedures under the supervision of an RN or physician. However, they have less autonomy and decision-making power than RNs.

To become an LPN, individuals must complete a state-approved practical nursing program, which typically takes about one year to complete. The program includes both classroom instruction and hands-on clinical training to prepare students for the demands of the job. After completing the program, LPNs must pass the National Council Licensure Examination (NCLEX-PN) to obtain licensure in their state. Some LPN programs may have additional education requirements, such as a high school diploma or equivalent. Overall, becoming an LPN requires less education and training than becoming an RN but still provides an important role in the healthcare industry.

Registered Nurse (RN)

Registered Nurses (RNs) are healthcare professionals who have completed a nursing program and obtained a nursing license. They can work in various settings, including hospitals, clinics, long-term care facilities, schools, and community centers. RNs have a broader scope of practice than LPNs and CNAs and are responsible for providing direct patient care, administering medications, performing diagnostic tests, and developing and implementing patient care plans. RNs also coordinate care with other healthcare professionals, such as physicians, nurse practitioners, and other members of the healthcare team.

To become an RN, individuals must complete an accredited nursing program, which can take anywhere from 2 to 4 years. A 2-year nursing degree grants an Associate Degree in Nursing (ADN), while a 4-year degree grants a Bachelor of Science in Nursing (BSN); however, both degrees grant the title of RN. Nursing programs typically include both classroom instruction and hands-on clinical training to prepare students for the demands of the job. After completing the program, RNs must pass the National Council Licensure Examination (NCLEX-RN) to obtain licensure in their state.

RNs also have the option of pursuing advanced degrees, such as a Master of Science in Nursing (MSN) or Doctor of Nursing Practice (DNP), which can lead to advanced practice roles and leadership positions within the healthcare industry. With their higher level of education and training compared to LPNs and CNAs, RNs are responsible for providing more advanced patient care.

Nurse Practitioner (NP)

Nurse Practitioners (NPs) are advanced practice registered nurses who have completed a Master of Science in Nursing (MSN) or Doctor of Nursing Practice (DNP) degree and obtained a nursing license. They have an expanded scope of practice beyond RNs and are authorized to provide a full range of healthcare services, including diagnosing and treating illnesses, prescribing medications, and ordering and interpreting diagnostic tests. NPs work collaboratively with physicians and other healthcare professionals to provide comprehensive patient care across lifespans.

To become an NP, individuals must first become a licensed RN and then complete a graduate-level nursing program that focuses on their chosen specialty. NP specialties include gerontology, psychiatric-mental health, women's health, and pediatrics, amongst others. NPs must also pass a national certification exam to obtain licensure in their state. Depending on the state, NPs may have full practice authority or may be required to work under the supervision of a physician. With their advanced education and training, NPs are able to provide high-quality care and play an important role in improving access to healthcare, particularly in underserved areas.

Certified Registered Nurse Anesthetist (CRNA)

Certified Registered Nurse Anesthetists (CRNAs) are advanced practice registered nurses who specialize in administering anesthesia to patients. They work in a variety of healthcare settings, including hospitals, surgical centers, and dental offices. CRNAs are responsible for assessing patients, determining the appropriate anesthesia dosage, and monitoring patients throughout the procedure to ensure their safety and comfort. They also manage patients' pain during and after surgical procedures and provide emergency care if needed.

To become a CRNA, individuals must first obtain a Bachelor of Science in Nursing (BSN) degree and become a licensed RN. They must then complete a Master of Science in Nursing (MSN) or a Doctorate of Nurse Practice (DNP) with a focus on anesthesia, which typically takes 2-3 years to complete. However, after 2025, new CRNAs must have a doctoral degree to enter the field, and an MSN will no longer be accepted.

After completing their education, CRNAs must pass a national certification exam and maintain ongoing education and training to maintain their certification. Due to their specialized training and expertise, CRNAs are among the highest-paid nursing professionals and are in high demand in the healthcare industry.

CHAPTER 3

HOW TO CHOOSE A NURSING PROGRAM

Choosing a nursing program is a critical decision for individuals who want to become a nurse. When selecting a nursing program, it's essential to consider factors such as its accreditation, cost, location, and reputation. It's crucial to research and compare multiple nursing programs before making a final decision to ensure that the program aligns with your career goals and aspirations. The following sections will explain some of the most key factors to consider when choosing a nursing program.

1. Degree Choice & Length

The first step to choosing a nursing program is selecting the nursing role you want to pursue. Each role, from a CNA to LPN to RN, comes with different responsibilities and working environments. Once you choose a role that appeals to you, that will dictate the program you look for. A CNA program can be completed within a few weeks to months, and an LPN program within a year. If you want to be an RN, the program can range from 2-4 years. ADN and BSN-prepared nurses can perform the same job duties, although BSN-prepared nurses have a more in-depth knowledge base, are better prepared for leadership roles, and have the opportunity to earn higher wages. In addition, some facilities require nurses to have a BSN.

Some nurses choose to earn an ADN first and pursue a BSN later. The benefit of this route is two-fold: some healthcare facilities have tuition reimbursement programs that may pay for some or all of the nurse's BSN program. Additionally, programs exist that allow ADN-prepared nurses to earn a BSN in as little as a year. Individuals with a bachelor's degree in another unrelated field have additional options as well. Many nursing programs around the country allow applicants with an existing bachelor's degree to earn a BSN in as little as 20 months. Overall, your preferred path will depend on your individual preferences and existing qualifications.

2. Location

When considering the location of a nursing school, there are several important factors to consider. First, is it within driving distance, or would you have to relocate? In addition to researching the cost of living in the area, you should also research the climate, culture, and overall quality of life there. Would you qualify for in-state or out-of-state tuition? How would you feel living away from your family or support system? All of these factors can have a significant impact on your experience while attending nursing school. Ultimately, you should consider all aspects of the school's location to ensure it's the right fit for your individual needs and preferences.

3. State Approval & Accreditation

When looking for prospective nursing programs, it's important to look at both state approval and program accreditation. State approval is mandatory, and a nursing program must have approval from the state's Board of Nursing in order to grant your license. This can be searched by navigating to the state's Board of Nursing website.

Although accreditation is not mandatory, attending a nursing program that is not accredited can cause major complications down the line. First, accreditation offers peace of mind that your program meets the quality standards established by the U.S. Department of Education. Beyond that, it allows students to easily receive financial aid, pursue advanced degrees, and obtain employment.

The two main accreditation bodies for U.S. nursing programs are The Accreditation Commission for Education in Nursing (ACEN) and The Commission on Collegiate Nursing Education (CCNE). It's also worth noting that although a school may be accredited, that doesn't automatically mean its nursing program is.

4. Tuition

Tuition is an important factor to consider when choosing a nursing school because it can significantly impact your financial situation. Nursing programs can vary in cost, and it's important to consider the tuition and other related expenses, such as textbooks, lab fees, and clinical fees, when making your decision. However, it's also important to keep in mind that a higher tuition doesn't necessarily mean a better education. Financial aid, grants, and scholarships are various ways to mitigate the out-of-cost expense of attending a nursing program. Additionally, especially due to the nursing shortage, programs like loan forgiveness and tuition reimbursement are quite common.

5. Class Structure & Size

When choosing a nursing program, it's important to consider the class structure. This includes whether the program offers online or in-person classes, the size of the classes, and the time spent in clinicals. Many nursing programs now offer online courses, which can provide more flexibility for students who may have other commitments, although some people learn better in a physical class with easier access to the instructor. Class size is also an important consideration, as smaller classes can allow for more personalized attention from instructors. At first glance, school size may not seem like an important factor to consider, but both have pros and cons. Larger schools, for example, may offer more resources and opportunities, while smaller schools may offer a more intimate learning environment.

Clinicals are also important to consider since they'll provide you with hands-on experience and exposure to the real-life situations you'll encounter as a nurse. This practical experience allows students to apply their theoretical knowledge in a clinical setting, gaining valuable skills in patient care, communication, critical thinking, and decision-making.

Some factors to consider when evaluating the clinicals of a nursing program include the variety and quality of clinical sites, the number of clinical hours required, and the level of support and guidance provided by clinical instructors. It is also important to consider the proximity of clinical sites to the nursing school and the availability of transportation options. Additionally, it may be helpful to research the types of patients and medical conditions that you'll have exposure to during your clinical rotations, as this can impact the breadth and depth of your clinical experience.

6. School Ratings & NCLEX Pass Rates

Next, look at the school's ratings and reputation within the healthcare industry. Factors such as accreditation, faculty qualifications, and student satisfaction can give you an idea of the program's quality and how it compares to other programs. You may also want to consider the school's overall reputation and the level of respect it commands from employers in the field. By choosing a highly-rated nursing program, you can increase your chances of receiving a high-quality education that prepares you for a successful career in nursing.

Another important factor to consider when choosing a nursing program is the school's NCLEX pass rates. The NCLEX is the national licensing exam for nurses, and passing it is required to obtain a nursing license. Nursing programs with high NCLEX pass rates typically have a strong curriculum and faculty, as well as effective student support services to help students succeed. By choosing a nursing program with a strong track record of NCLEX pass rates, you will receive a quality education that prepares you for success on this critical exam and in your nursing career.

As an aspiring nurse, you need to select a nursing program that aligns with your goals, especially since the choice of a nursing program can impact everything from your finances to your employability and future career opportunities. It can be overwhelming to consider all the factors when choosing a nursing program, but some strategies can make the process more manageable.

One effective approach is to get organized and create a plan. This might involve writing out all the factors to consider, such as program location, clinical opportunities, class structure, and tuition costs. It's also important to stay organized with entry deadlines, requirements, and any additional costs such as textbooks or fees. Creating a spreadsheet or checklist is another helpful tool for keeping track of all the pertinent information. By getting organized and considering all the relevant factors, you can make an informed decision about the nursing program that best aligns with your goals and needs, setting you up for long-term success!

CHAPTER 4

PREPARATION & PREREQUISITES

Preparing to apply to nursing school involves careful planning and attention to detail. One of the first steps is to review the academic requirements of the nursing programs being considered. Typically, nursing schools require applicants to have a high school diploma or equivalent, and some may require specific courses such as biology, chemistry, and anatomy and physiology. It is important that you carefully review these requirements and ensure all prerequisites are met. Additionally, some nursing programs may require applicants to have a minimum GPA or specific grades in prerequisite courses.

Getting into nursing school is a competitive process, and you must put in your best effort to increase your chances of acceptance. It's important to strive for excellence and never do the bare minimum! Simply meeting the minimum requirements may not be enough, so you should always aim to go above and beyond to demonstrate your commitment and dedication.

Another important consideration is the entrance exams required by many nursing programs. The Test of Essential Academic Skills (TEAS) or the Health Education Systems, Inc. (HESI) exams are commonly used to assess an applicant's knowledge and aptitude in areas such as reading comprehension, math, and science. Preparing for these exams can be critical in the application process.

Some nursing programs may require or prefer applicants to have previous healthcare experience, such as working as a certified nursing assistant (CNA) or medical assistant. This can demonstrate to the admissions committee that the applicant has experience in the field and a strong understanding of the job demands. Even if work experience is not required for entry, having healthcare experience can still give you an advantage. Admissions committees may view applicants with healthcare experience as having a clearer understanding of what it means to be a nurse and as being more prepared for the rigors of nursing school. Additionally, applicants with prior healthcare experience have the chance to work with patients and get hands-on experience, which can help students understand the nursing courses in a deeper way.

Some nursing programs require letters of recommendation as part of the application process. These letters can come from previous teachers, employers, or healthcare professionals who can attest to your character, work ethic, and aptitude for the nursing profession. It is important to carefully select individuals who can provide a strong endorsement and submit these letters in accordance with the school's instructions.

Other possible requirements include submitting transcripts, test scores, essays, and other materials, with each school having its own specific requirements. It's important to review these requirements carefully and ensure that all materials are submitted on time. Double and triple-check the instructions before submitting anything!

If you're worried about some aspect of your application, don't worry—it can be comforting to know that most nursing schools evaluate applicants by compiling a total score based on multiple metrics rather than focusing on a single metric. Factors such as GPA, ACT or SAT scores, math and science grades, letters of recommendation, personal statements, and interviews are all taken into consideration. By looking at a range of factors, nursing schools can gain a complete picture of each applicant and their potential as a future nurse. This approach also allows for greater flexibility in admissions decisions, as a lower GPA may be offset by strong performance in other areas, such as work experience or an exceptional interview.

When applying, start early and stay organized. Make a list of deadlines and application materials needed for each program. Be sure to review the application instructions carefully and submit all required materials on time. It's also a good idea to apply to multiple nursing programs to increase your chances of acceptance. However, it's still important to research each program thoroughly and ensure it aligns with your educational and career goals before applying. Many schools have application fees, and applying to several programs can be expensive, so budget accordingly. But ultimately, applying to multiple nursing programs can be a strategic way to increase your chances of acceptance and give you more options to choose from.

In conclusion, applying to nursing school requires careful planning and attention to detail. While the process may be competitive and time-consuming, you need to remain positive and remember why you wanted to pursue nursing in the first place. With perseverance and a strong work ethic, you can achieve your dream of becoming a registered nurse and make a positive impact in the healthcare field!

CHAPTER 5

READY, SET, INTERVIEW: MASTERING THE NURSING SCHOOL ADMISSIONS PROCESS

You've been granted an interview—congratulations on making it this far! Although preparing for a nursing school interview can be a nerve-wracking experience, it's important to remember that the interview is an opportunity to showcase your strengths and demonstrate why you are a good fit for the program. To prepare, research the program and familiarize yourself with the school's mission, values, and curriculum.

It's also important to dress professionally, wearing conservative business attire and minimal accessories. Arrive early to avoid traffic or any unforeseen circumstance that could make you late—this also gives you extra time to gather your thoughts and relax before the interview. Bringing a resume and other supporting materials is always a good idea as well, such as a copy of your resume or transcripts.

During the interview, listen carefully to the questions being asked and take your time when answering. Try to provide specific examples and experiences to support your answers and ask follow-up questions if needed. To decrease your anxiety, it can be really helpful to practice interviewing with a friend or family member. Formulating your answers out loud (especially when you're nervous!) is great practice for the real interview. Some common interview questions you may encounter are:

• What are your strengths and weaknesses?

It's important to be honest and thoughtful when answering this common interview question. For strengths, highlight qualities that are valuable in a nursing student and future nurse, such as empathy, compassion, strong communication skills, attention to detail, and a willingness to learn. When discussing weaknesses, avoid making excuses or being overly critical of oneself. Instead, focus on areas where improvement is needed and demonstrate a plan for addressing those weaknesses. For example, a weakness might be a lack of experience in a specific area of healthcare, but the applicant could discuss plans to gain experience through volunteering or shadowing. Ultimately, the key is to demonstrate self-awareness, a willingness to learn and improve, and a positive attitude toward personal growth.

- **What can you bring to the program? Why should the school/program choose you amongst the other applicants?**

To answer this question, try to highlight your unique strengths and experiences that will benefit the program. You can discuss your passion for nursing and your dedication to helping others. Share your experiences working in healthcare, volunteering at hospitals or clinics, or participating in nursing-related activities. Highlight your skills and how they can be applied to nursing, such as strong communication skills, attention to detail, or the ability to work well under pressure.

You can also mention any special talents or qualities that set you apart from other applicants, such as bilingualism, cultural awareness, or leadership experience. Be confident and concise in your response, and try to connect your strengths and experiences to how they will contribute to the nursing program and, most importantly, how those skills will benefit patients.

- **Why do you want to become a nurse?**

When answering this question, there are few wrong answers, as long as the student communicates a genuine passion for the profession and a desire to make a positive impact. It's helpful to draw upon personal experiences or connections to healthcare that sparked the student's interest in nursing. Additionally, emphasizing the desire to constantly learn and improve, as well as the dedication to teamwork and collaboration, can demonstrate applicable strengths to becoming a nurse. Overall, being authentic, passionate, and thoughtful in your answer can make a strong impression on the interviewer and showcase your potential as a future nurse.

• **Why did you choose this program/school?**

Before the interview, take time to review the program's website and mission statement to understand its values and goals. Consider how the program aligns with your own personal and career goals. Select a few aspects of the program or school that attracted you, such as its curriculum, clinical opportunities, faculty, or community partnerships. Show your enthusiasm and passion for the program, and be authentic in your response. Finally, connect your answer back to the ways in which you feel the program will help you become the best nurse you can be.

In addition to asking personal questions to gain insight into your personality, communication skills, and ability to work with others, there may also be situational questions related to how you would handle certain clinical scenarios. These questions are designed to assess the applicant's critical thinking skills and ability to make sound decisions under pressure. Some of the questions may include:

- **How would you handle a difficult patient?**

When answering this question, try to demonstrate your ability to remain calm and empathetic in challenging situations. You should describe how you would use effective communication techniques to try and understand the patient's concerns and work towards a resolution. It's important to emphasize the importance of building trust and rapport with patients to create a positive working relationship. Try to mention your understanding of the importance of maintaining professional boundaries and seeking assistance from supervisors or colleagues if needed. Providing specific examples of similar situations you've experienced and how you handled them can also strengthen your answer.

• How would you handle a disagreement with a doctor or colleague?

Emphasize the importance of open communication and a team approach to patient care. One strategy could be to discuss the importance of actively listening to the other party's perspective and trying to understand their point of view. Additionally, highlighting the importance of remaining calm and professional during a conflict and trying to find a mutually beneficial solution could be helpful. It's also important to discuss the value of seeking guidance from a supervisor or mentor if the situation can't be resolved independently. Ultimately, the key is to demonstrate a willingness to work collaboratively and prioritize the patient's needs above personal conflicts.

When the interview draws to a close, the interviewer may ask if you have any questions. Although it may be tempting to say "no" and run out of there, take advantage of this opportunity to learn more about the program and show your interest. Come prepared with a few thoughtful questions about the program, such as the curriculum, clinical opportunities, or student support services. You can also ask about the interviewer's experience in the nursing field or any advice they may have for a prospective nursing student. By asking thoughtful questions, you can demonstrate your enthusiasm for the program and show that you have done your research.

In addition to being prepared, it's also important to be honest and authentic. Remember that the nursing school interview process is a two-way street, and it's also an opportunity to evaluate whether the program is the right fit for you. After the interview, following up with a thank-you email or note can also make a positive impression. By using these tips and strategies, you can feel confident and well-prepared for the interview process and set yourself up for a successful nursing career.

CHAPTER 6

NURSING SCHOOL SURVIVAL GUIDE: TIPS AND STRATEGIES FOR SUCCEEDING IN YOUR PROGRAM

Congratulations! You nailed the interview, and you've been accepted into nursing school. Now the real work begins. This final chapter will provide you with valuable tips and strategies to help you succeed in your nursing program. These suggestions will help you manage your time effectively, reduce stress, and develop critical skills necessary for a successful nursing career.

Time Management

Time management is particularly critical in nursing school due to the demanding nature of the curriculum, which often includes a combination of rigorous coursework, clinical rotations, and preparation for licensure exams. Balancing these responsibilities requires careful planning and organization to ensure that you're able to meet deadlines, adequately prepare for exams, and develop the practical skills necessary for your future nursing career.

Additionally, effective time management is essential for reducing stress and preventing burnout, which is common among nursing students due to the high-pressure environment and expectations. By managing your time wisely, you can create a more balanced schedule that allows for regular study sessions, breaks, and self-care activities, ultimately contributing to a healthier and more sustainable nursing school experience.

By developing strong time management skills during nursing school, you'll also benefit your future self. As a nurse, you'll be responsible for managing multiple tasks, prioritizing patient care, and making quick decisions in fast-paced, high-stakes situations. By mastering time management now, you'll be better prepared to excel as a professional nurse and provide quality care to your patients. Here are some tips to help you stay on top of your schedule:

- Use a planner or calendar to track assignments, exams, and clinical rotations.

- Break down large tasks into smaller, manageable steps.

- Prioritize tasks based on importance and deadlines.

- Schedule regular study time and avoid procrastination.

- Allow for breaks and relaxation to prevent burnout.

Develop Effective Study Habits

Developing effective study habits enhances your ability to understand complex nursing concepts, leading to improved academic performance and, ultimately, success in taking the NCLEX! These habits also lay the foundation for lifelong professional growth, ensuring that you can adapt to advances in healthcare and provide high-quality patient care. Furthermore, effective study habits contribute to better stress management and overall well-being, helping to avoid last-minute cramming and exam anxiety. Consider the following study tips:

- Attend all classes and take thorough notes.

- Review lecture material and assigned readings regularly.

- Form a study group with classmates to discuss course material and share insights.

- Utilize additional resources, such as online forums, textbooks, and even YouTube videos.

- Practice critical thinking and problem-solving skills through case studies and simulations.

Stay Organized

Nursing school is even more demanding than other programs since it involves both classes and clinicals. Getting (and staying) organized is essential to making your life easier and ensuring you stay on track. Keep track of important documents, assignments, and course materials by:

- Organizing your notes and study materials by subject or course.

- Regularly updating your planner or calendar with important dates and tasks.

- Backing up digital files to avoid losing important documents.

- Accurately record the dates, times, and locations of clinical sites.

Build a Support Network

Nursing school is tough! Building a support network is vital, as it provides a foundation of encouragement, motivation, and shared knowledge during the challenging journey. A strong support network consisting of peers, instructors, and mentors fosters collaboration and allows you to exchange insights, discuss course material, and seek guidance when faced with obstacles. Additionally, you can form lasting relationships that will not only enhance your nursing school experience but also contribute to your long-term success and personal growth in your nursing career. Some ways you can connect with peers, instructors, and mentors is by:

- Participating in class discussions and engaging with classmates.

- Attending study groups, workshops, and nursing-related events.

- Joining professional nursing organizations and online forums.

- Seeking guidance from instructors and mentors when facing challenges.

Maintain a Healthy Balance

Maintaining a healthy balance is critical in nursing school because it will help you manage stress, prevent burnout, and remain focused on your academic and professional goals. By prioritizing self-care, you'll take care of your mental and physical well-being, which directly impacts your performance in class and clinical settings. Equally as important as self-care is having fun! Setting aside time for hobbies and interests outside of nursing school will allow you to recharge and maintain a sense of perspective, ultimately contributing to a more positive, sustainable, and fulfilling educational experience. Take care of yourself by:

- Eating a balanced diet and staying hydrated.

- Getting regular exercise and practicing stress-relief techniques, such as meditation or yoga.

- Prioritizing sleep and maintaining a consistent sleep schedule.

- Making time for hobbies and interests outside of nursing school.

Embrace Clinical Rotations

Clinical rotations are hands-on practice for the real job duties you'll be performing as a nurse. Clinicals are invaluable since they offer a safe space to practice your skills under the guidance of an expert. Ask questions and soak up these experiences as much as you can—you'll be glad to draw on these experiences later. Additionally, clinical instructors are full of knowledge and are happy to walk you through new and nerve-wracking situations. To make the most of these experiences:

- Arrive prepared and punctual for each clinical shift.

- Be proactive in seeking opportunities to practice new skills.

- Ask questions and learn from experienced nurses and other healthcare professionals.

- Reflect on your experiences and identify areas for improvement.

Prepare for Exams and Licensing

Ultimately, nursing school is preparation for two things: the NCLEX and your future career as a nurse. By consistently reviewing course material and utilizing NCLEX-RN study resources throughout nursing school, you can not only increase your likelihood of passing the licensing exam but improve your performance in classes. To prepare for these challenges:

- Review course material consistently throughout the semester.

- Utilize NCLEX-RN study resources and practice exams.

- Attend review courses or workshops.

- Stay informed about licensing requirements and application deadlines.

This short e-book is designed to provide you with valuable insights and friendly advice to help you thrive during your exciting nursing school journey. Although nursing school is challenging, it's a pursuit that is well worth it! When you're struggling, remember the end goal—a rewarding career, financial freedom, and, most importantly, the chance to positively impact people's lives. Embrace these tips and strategies with confidence, and remember that you're on your way to becoming an incredible nurse who will make a real difference in the lives of your patients and the communities you serve. You've got this!

ABOUT THE AUTHOR

Nekesha Johnson is a Registered Nurse from Grenada, Mississippi. With 8 years of experience in the nursing field, she has worked in a wide range of specialties, from medical surgery and pediatrics to orthopedics and oncology. Nekesha earned her Associate Degree in Nursing from Holmes Community College, followed by a Bachelor's Degree and a Master of Science in Nursing from Mississippi University for Women. As a proud mother of her daughter, Na'La Meon Tidwell, Nekesha cherishes her time outside of work. She enjoys exploring the world through travel and embracing her adventurous side.

Driven by a passion for helping others, Nekesha wrote this e-book to provide a clear and concise blueprint for aspiring nursing students who may lack guidance in pursuing their dreams. Often, academic advisors may inadvertently guide students to take non-essential classes or follow an inefficient course plan, which can delay the realization of their dream to become a nurse. Through her personal experiences and expertise, Nekesha aims to empower future nurses with the knowledge and tools they need to succeed in their nursing education and careers.